Going Gentle Into That Good Night:

A Practical and Informative Guide For Fulfilling the Circle of Life For Our Loved Ones with Dementias and Alzheimer's Disease

By Sandra Ross

©2013

Table of Contents

Do Not Go Gentle Into That Good Night

Do not go gentle into that good night,
Old age should burn and rave at close of day;
Rage, rage against the dying of the light.

Though wise men at their end know dark is right,
Because their words had forked no lightning they
Do not go gentle into that good night.

Good men, the last wave by, crying how bright
Their frail deeds might have danced in a green
bay,
Rage, rage against the dying of the light.

Wild men who caught and sang the sun in flight,
And learn, too late, they grieved it on its way,
Do not go gentle into that good night.

Grave men, near death, who see with blinding
sight
Blind eyes could blaze like meteors and be gay,
Rage, rage against the dying of the light.

And you, my father, there on that sad height,
Curse, bless, me now with your fierce tears, I
pray.
Do not go gentle into that good night.
Rage, rage against the dying of the light.

Dylan Thomas

Chapter 1: Warning Signs

After my dad's death in 1998, I stepped into his shoes - although it was impossible to fill them - as my mom's primary protector, resource manager, and advisor. I had promised my dad I would take care of her in our last face-to-face conversation before his death, and I was committed to fulfilling that promise.

Of the three of us kids, I had always been the one who maintained the closest relationship with my parents. My other siblings had jobs and lives that, after they left home, inevitably took over as their priorities and focus, and Dad and Mom, while in the picture, moved out of their primary lines of vision.

I always had a sense of the circle of life and my need to step into the role with them and for them that they had provided for us growing up as I saw them age and start struggling with serious health issues.

My dad battled congestive heart failure for ten years, the last year of which was brutal for him in terms of suffering. Although I miss him and always will until I see him again, I am thankful that his suffering is over.

Mom, as she worked toward acceptance of the huge void my dad's death left in her heart and her life, began to cling to me the way she had to my dad, not in a dependent way, but as backup and security. Mom made me her medical power of attorney within a month after Dad's death.

Despite her grief and the almost insurmountable adjustment to life without her soul mate, Mom began to get busy doing what her life's work was about: continuing to learn and grow as many new things as she was able and helping other people.

For the next six years, she flourished and despite a few health issues – skin cancer was the most serious – she remained active and vibrant and alert and curious, as she had been all her life.

She was an avid walker and, when I moved to Tennessee in 2004, to be close to her, we enjoyed walking every day together. She could not walk the distances I could, but she did very well for her age.

In 2005, the faint warning signs of change started emerging. Mom had always been a multitasker and, because of that, somewhat ADD, but it seemed to get more pronounced in 2005.

She'd had TIA's - anxiety-induced - all her life, but I noticed them happening with more regular frequency. Her blood pressure was always problematic, but never outside of acceptable ranges, so I knew that the TIA's were a result of some kind of internal anxiety she was dealing with.

Although Mom was a talker, she never told - or maybe just didn't know how to tell me - me what was causing her to be anxious. I tried to keep things on an even keel and stay calm when she was in obvious high anxiety mode, and sometimes I was able to calm her down and sometimes not.

In the early summer of 2005, Mom decided to create a revocable trust with her as the trustee and me as the trustee in the event that she became incapacitated or died.

With the trust, she retained sole control over her legal and financial matters (while I helped her with banking and legal matters, I had no access to do anything with her bank accounts and I had no legal power over her affairs).

She did this because, in her words, "since you're taking care of me, I want to make sure if I have anything left, it goes to you."

I reminded her at this point, as I had in all our previous conversations and all the ones subsequent to this one, that Dad had left everything to her. It was for her. I told her that if the check I wrote to the funeral home bounced because she'd been taken care of then we'd be all right.

There was a period in the late summer of 2005 when Mom was often dizzy and felt faint and we made a few trips to the ER and had one hospital admission. There didn't seem to be any cause that the doctors were able to identify, but by the fall, the symptoms had gone away.

There were a couple of incidents that were more major warning signs, however, that I didn't recognize at the time.

Mom had a profound hearing loss all her life and as she got older, it got more pronounced. Initially, when we started having "misunderstandings," I believed it was because she heard something different than what I said, so I'd try to explain it more clearly to make sure she understood, with mixed results.

Mom also, because of a very traumatic childhood, had always had back notes of fear, paranoia, and suspiciousness about what other people were doing and why. Her biggest fear, because it happened in her childhood, was that people were stealing from her or taking what belonged to her.

I think the hearing loss exacerbated these back notes and during and after 2005, they became much more pronounced.

The first incident was a speeding ticket that Mom got. She was going 40 mph in a 35 mph zone. I believe this was the only ticket Mom ever got in all the years she drove.

I have no doubt that the traffic cop was a jerk because I talked to someone whose husband was also a policeman and she said there had been a lot of complaints about this officer.

But Mom was livid. As she recounted the incident to me when I got home from work, she said he treated her like a criminal. Because of that, after she got the ticket, she went straight to the police department and reported him and tried to get them to void the ticket.

They would not. Her only option was to go to a defensive driving class if she didn't want to pay the fine and have the ticket go against her license.

Mom ended up going to the class, but she was still very angry about the whole incident and talked about it incessantly.

The second thing that happened was more puzzling to me. We had started discussing me buying a house closer to town for the two of us so that she was close to all the places she went and the things that she was involved in.

Somehow she came away from these discussions with the idea that I wanted her to buy the house (I did not - I had the income and credit score to afford to buy) and "use up all her money."

No matter how many times I corrected her, as long as she was able to remember, that was her version of these conversations. And because that was her version, she, without my knowledge, decided to move into an independent living retirement community.

I found this out when I got home from work one day and she announced that she was moving and had already signed the paperwork and made the deposits.

I was surprised and asked why. Somehow it all got turned around on me that I didn't want her around and she'd be out of my way.

Again, I futilely tried to set the record straight, but she'd already convinced herself of her perception of things, so I was never successful in clearing things up.

Once she'd done that, though, I began to look for a place to buy near where she was living, so I could be there at a moment's notice when she needed me. I found a condo less than a mile away, bought it and told her I'd be by to see her every day and to spend time with her, and, with very few exceptions, I was.

She seemed happier and calmer after moving. Mom was an extrovert and she liked being around people, so the community atmosphere suited her. She got involved in activities there and continued the activities she enjoyed outside of the community as well.

We established a routine where she would come over to my place on Fridays, do her laundry and mine, and she'd clean up downstairs. I didn't need her to do any of that, but when I told her she didn't have to, she got upset. She complained that I wouldn't let her do anything for me, so I told her if that made her happy, then I'd appreciate her doing it. I'd pick her up on Friday evenings after work and take her out for a nice dinner, which we both enjoyed.

2006 came and went without many warning signs. The few that appeared were so far apart that I didn't connect them. One thing I did notice was her physically slowing down toward the end of the year. She'd had an aortic valve replacement in 1994 that had a 10-year guarantee on it, so I figured that was beginning to wear out. She remained active, but when we traveled, she was not able to walk even slowly for several hours, as we'd always done in the past.

2007 had a few incidents that gave me pause, but I still wasn't adding them up because they were, again, scattered throughout the year.

The first was in late January. I was working a little later than usual on a frigid night. I had called Mom to tell her I'd drop by after I finished the project I was working on and she was panicky on the phone.

Mom told me that she'd hit something on the way home - she didn't know what - and the window was broken on the front passenger door.

I told Mom I'd get something on the way to her place to protect it and we'd take it to get it fixed the next morning and get her a rental car while it was being fixed.

When I got to Mom's place, her panic was full-blown anxiety. I went out to the parking lot with Mom and was alarmed to see that the whole passenger door was damaged badly.

I didn't say anything to Mom, because I knew she was already upset, but I was terrified that she had side-swiped a car unknowingly and we'd be getting charges for Mom leaving the scene of an accident and her license would be taken away.

I alerted a couple of close friends to what had happened, since I was leaving town for a funeral that Friday and wouldn't be back until Monday afternoon. The next morning, we got the car in to be repaired and I got Mom into a rental car.

While I was gone, the couple I'd alerted - and whom Mom trusted - visited Mom and asked her to show them where the damage to the car had happened.

Mom took them to a road where there were no parked cars allowed, but a fairly high curb, so the husband concluded that Mom must have sideswiped the curb by overcorrecting the car for some reason.

I figured that was reasonable and didn't warrant considering the possibility that Mom needed to stop driving.

There were a few falls at my house when Mom was there on Fridays that year as well, one of which resulted in a wrist injury, but nothing more serious.

I was getting concerned, though, about her balance in general, but since overall she was still active and moving pretty well most of the time, I kept it on a back burner.

2008 was the beginning of more frequent and urgent warning signs. At the time, I did not realize the sum total of them, so I share this with you so you can benefit from my experiences.

The first thing materialized early in the year.

Suddenly Mom was unable to get appointments with an internist that she'd been seeing for several years.

According to Mom, the nurses would not call her back and even when she went into the office, they ignored her. Mom wanted to change doctors.

I suggested another internist in that group, but she didn't want to do that because she was worried that her previous internist would be upset and that she'd still have trouble getting appointments.

So I found another group and another internist and I began going to Mom's doctor appointments with her.

Mom didn't like the internist I chose because he was abrupt and he wouldn't listen to her. Although the internist's "bedside manner" was indeed horrible, I knew that part of the problem was that Mom would ramble randomly about everything medically and would not - it never occurred to me that Mom could not - focus on the purpose for the visit.

I could see both of them getting more irritated with each other with each successive visit. I began then advocating for Mom with the doctor. At times, Mom was okay with this and at times she was not, but I realized immediate issues were not going to be addressed if I didn't.

Beginning in late March of that year, Mom's blood pressure began to spike uncontrollably on a frequent basis.

Mom also was having more frequent bowel impactions and upset stomachs that resulted in profuse vomiting.

By late May, Mom and I were frequent visitors each week to the ER, mostly because of Mom's elevated blood pressure.

Mom's internist seemed unconcerned with the blood pressure spikes and made no changes to her medicine.

As June wore on, we were at the ER nightly because of Mom's blood pressure spikes. The staff would get them under control and send us home.

Finally in late June, after yet another ER trip, the ER doctor suspected that Mom had a blood clot somewhere, and he admitted her.

I made a quick trip to Mom's place to get a bag of clothes and toiletries packed for her (after this hospital admission, I kept a packed bag at Mom's place with all these items in them, so I could take it with us when we went to the hospital), and then came back to spend the night, which I generally did when Mom was in the hospital.

The next day brought ultrasounds and the confirmation that Mom had two lung embolisms. The treatment included rest and medications, including heparin shots, to break up the clots before they could dislodge and go to her brain and cause a stroke.

By week's end, Mom was feeling better, but was still very weak and tired. On Saturday, she had a series of TIA's and we went by ambulance to a larger hospital for another embolism scan. There were none, but her doctor at the hospital decided to keep Mom for another week to get her strength up and slowly get her back into normal activity.

When Mom was released, one of the medications she had to take was the blood thinner Coumadin.

With that came the weekly INR blood work, the dosage adjustments - which I kept up with because it was clear Mom wasn't going to be able to handle something changing that often - and the limitations on what Mom could eat (green leafy vegetables, which both Mom and I really liked, have a lot of Vitamin K, which can lower the effectiveness of Coumadin).

After about a month of this, Mom and I were taking a walk one Friday afternoon and Mom told me she was ready to die and she simply did not want to have to take all these medications and go through all the blood work involved.

I said, "Okay. I'll call the doctor Monday and have him taper you off of it."

Her internist protested, but I explained that this what Mom wanted and, as her medical power of attorney, I was going to honor her wishes.

Reluctantly, he stopped the Coumadin, but at the one appointment we had with him after that, his attitude toward Mom was disrespectful and he clearly couldn't be bothered with her.

Mom was justifiably very upset after the appointment. I was upset too.

I told Mom that I thought it was time to find a good general practice physician who could refer her to specialists, if need be, but who would be interested in her general health and well-being.

Mom agreed. I quickly managed to find a physician's assistant who specialized in geriatric medicine to take her as a patient.

He and Mom fell in love with each other at the first appointment. He listened patiently to Mom's spiel of randomness and asked a lot of questions and actually listened to her answers.

He showed Mom a lot of respect and was not condescending or arrogant with her.

I was happy and Mom was happy and it was a good decision at that time.

The weekly ER trips for Mom's high blood pressure started again around the beginning of August.

The last week of August, we made another night trip to the ER. Over several hours the staff tried to get Mom's blood pressure lowered and it was not coming down.

I told the ER doctor that they needed to admit Mom because I wasn't comfortable with the amount of medicine they'd given her with no measurable results.

The ER doctor said they'd give one more dose and one more hour and if Mom's blood pressure wasn't lower, they'd admit her.

Within an hour, Mom's blood pressure was down to high normal. The ER doctor said they were not going to admit her.

I told the ER doctor I thought it was a bad idea because they'd given Mom so much medicine to get her blood pressure down to high normal and it still was not in optimal range.

The ER doctor said they were discharging Mom anyway. I noted on the discharge papers my concern and that I disagreed with the discharge.

By then, it was after 3 a.m. Mom was wiped out. I got Mom home and ready for bed and tucked her in before leaving around 4:30 a.m. I got home, started coffee, and got ready for work.

About 9:30 that morning, I got a call from the nursing staff where Mom lived and the nurse told me that Mom's blood pressure was really low – she'd tried to get up and was weak and dizzy – and I needed to get her to the hospital.

I left work immediately and got Mom back to the same ER we'd left just a few hours before.

The ER got Mom in right away and on monitors and not only was her blood pressure really low, but her heart rate was very slow.

I explained what had happened just a few hours before and the doctor said that Mom should have been admitted and not discharged. He told us that he was going to admit Mom to see what was going on.

I went home to get Mom's DNR and living will and within the short period of time it took for me to go and come back, Mom's heart rate had gone so low that the staff administered a heart stimulant and put Mom in ICU.

My first piece of advice is that you need to make sure you always have a copy of DNRs and living wills with you. Shortly after this, I had both reduced to 3"x5" size and kept them in an envelope in the console of my car.

This works out well for you, especially in emergency situations, like this one, when your loved ones are still independent to some extent. Once you become the sole advocate for them, keep an updated list of medications and dosages, daily vital signs, and a copy of all power of attorney documents, as well as DNRs and living wills in a backpack. Take the backpack everywhere, because you'll never know when you're going to need it.

Mom was resting quietly in ICU when I got back and I told her I was going to leave for a couple of hours to do some things I needed to get done for myself and her and I'd be back.

By the time I got back to Mom, she was restless and agitated. One problem was that she hadn't eaten all day. Even though her blood pressure and heart rate were still very low, she was animated and hungry. I managed to get Mom some food, but when it came, she was suspicious of it and angry at me because it wasn't something else.

The longer I was there, the more agitated Mom seemed to get, so I decided the best thing for both of us was for me to leave and come back the next morning.

I spoke to one of the ICU nurses on my way out and mentioned Mom's agitation and she said that was common in elderly people in the hospital, but they could have the doctor prescribe anti-anxiety medication for Mom.

I specifically asked that it be something mild and a low dose in light of the blood pressure and heart issues. The nurse assured me that was what she would ask the doctor to do.

About 6:30 the next morning, one of the ICU nurses called me and told me Mom had been out of control all night and I needed to get there right away.

I had been up for a couple hours and was ready to leave the house, so I was at the hospital five minutes later. By the time I got there, Mom was calm, seemed glad to see me, but didn't know exactly why she was there or what was going on.

I held Mom's hand and explained everything. As I explained, I could see the light of remembrance of the events of the past couple of days come on in Mom's eyes.

Mom squeezed my hand and told me she was glad I was there. I told her I wasn't going anywhere and I'd be with her every step of the way.

A cardiologist came in around 7:30 a.m. and started asking Mom questions about her heart.

Mom's answers made no sense to him and no sense to me, so I started answering for her, and he decided they would do some heart tests (she was diagnosed with congestive heart failure, which would, as it had with my dad, be the physical condition that eventually worsened and contributed to Mom's death). Just minutes later, though, Mom didn't even remember the cardiologist being there.

By 9 a.m., my sister had arrived. We sat with Mom and talked with her. Around 9:30 a.m., she said the nurses were all having a party at the desk and eating cake.

My sister and I looked toward the desk and no one was there. We then instinctively looked at other and we both sort of shrugged, unsure what to do with that information.

However, from that point on, for the rest of the day – except for a bout of anger directed toward my sister during lunch – Mom talked incessantly about all the parties at the desk and everybody eating cake, the plane crashes she was seeing out there, the animals she was seeing out there, and the fun it looked like everyone was having out there.

In the middle of the afternoon, Mom started tracing letters in the air and asking my sister and me if we could read them. By now, we had no idea what was going on, but simply went along with Mom. We asked Mom to tell us what they said. She "read" them to us and was quite content and quite happy.

My sister and I always refer to this day as Mom's "Wizard of Oz" day, because it was the most bizarre, though not unpleasant on the whole, behavior we'd ever seen in Mom to that point.

By evening, though, right around dinnertime, Mom got angry and agitated again and my sister and I decided to leave and give Mom a chance to rest. We'd come back early the next morning.

I told the ICU nurse at the desk that Mom was pretty agitated and she said they had an anti-anxiety medicine ordered by the doctor and they'd give it to her.

In hindsight, I can only conclude that they must have given Mom a very large dose of the anti-anxiety medication that night, because when my sister and I got there early the next morning, Mom was totally unresponsive. Her heart rate and blood pressure were even lower than the day before.

Mom had a few lucid periods during the day where she told us she was ready to be with Daddy, but she did not eat or drink anything all day long, and was "asleep" most of the day.

We both believed Mom was dying.

But, as with the two previous evenings, right around dinner time, Mom was wide awake and very angry.

This time I got the brunt of it.

Mom loudly accused me of putting her in a nursing home without even discussing it with her. I told her Mom was in the hospital ICU because she had heart and blood pressure problems.

Mom then, just as loudly, called me a liar and got really nasty. I could not reason with Mom or convince her that what she believed wasn't true.

I was exasperated and decided the only thing that might help would be to get

Mom transferred to a regular room. If it was her time to go, then it really wouldn't matter whether she was in ICU or not.

I managed to convince the ICU nurse to move Mom to a regular patient room – which did calm her down some – and after I got her tucked in for the night, I got into the other bed in the room and spent the rest of the night trying to figure out what in the world was going on.

The next morning, Mom was lucid, but very weak, but seemed glad my sister and I were there. Mom had been catheterized in ICU and I noticed that morning that her urine was very concentrated, so I found a nurse and asked her if we could get Mom on a hydration IV because I realized that dehydration might be causing the symptoms we were seeing.

The nurse said she would get one started.

By 11 a.m., the IV had still not been started. Two nurses came in to get Mom washed up and dressed. They asked my sister and I to leave the room. We were standing just outside the half-open door when we heard a commotion in the room.

When we went into the room, we found the nurses struggling to hold Mom up and get her back in bed. We helped and I noticed as I was sat on the bed and held Mom's hand that her breathing was shallow, her blood pressure and heart rate were very low, and once again, I believed she was close to dying.

I asked again for the hydration IV. By now a doctor was in the room as well and she started pressing me to give medications to keep Mom alive.

Those were not Mom's wishes, so I told her that the only thing I would allow was the hydration IV. If that was not the problem and it was Mom's time to go, then I was going to honor her wishes.

The doctor kept pressing me to do more while the nurse was hooking up the IV and I kept refusing. Mom squeezed my hand and said again she was ready to be with Daddy.

I told Mom it was okay for her to go and that I loved her.

Mom closed her eyes. As she began to get hydrated, her breathing normalized and color began returning to her face. By early afternoon, Mom was awake and talking calmly and lucidly.

There were another couple of incidents during this stay in which Mom accused me of putting her in a mental institution and she got really nasty with my sister again, but for the most part, she was fairly lucid and fairly calm the rest of the stay.

When Mom was discharged a few days later, one of the nurses who'd been in the room when the doctor was pressing me to do what Mom didn't want done told me that Mom was about thirty seconds away from dying, but I made the right call and she admired my calmness and strength and respect for Mom's wishes in spite of all the chaos going on around me in that moment.

At this point in time, I believed Mom's most serious issues were heart and blood pressure and those were what I focused on in her care and medication.

Somehow, and this is a lesson learned, I managed to put aside the other infrequent mental/emotional issues Mom was exhibiting or explain them away in terms of blood flow (heart and blood pressure).

It never occurred to me then that these were warning signs I needed to bring to the forefront of my focus.

Admittedly, it was because these warning signs were sporadic, short-lived, and Mom was pretty okay most of the time. I knew people had "moments" as they aged and so because it wasn't constant or severe, I chalked it up to being part of the aging process.

The lesson? Don't overlook or ignore these early warning signs. While they may not be pervasive and life-changing at first, early treatment can help lessen the impact on your loved ones and you and give them a much higher and better quality of life for a longer duration.

After that hospital stay, Mom managed to stay out of the hospital, except for a couple of bowel impactions, for the rest of the year.

However, there were still these "flares" of warning signs that happened sporadically through the end of the year.

Thanksgiving stands out as one of those. My sister came into town for the long weekend. Mom and I had a tradition of going to a really nice buffet at one of the local hotels each Thanksgiving we were in town and it was just the two of us, so I'd made reservations for the three of us there mid-afternoon Thanksgiving Day.

My sister and I went over to pick Mom up mid-morning and bring her back to my house to play games and spend together before we went to eat.

All was fine and good until about a half hour before we were going to leave. Mom's disposition changed instantly and she was angry at both my sister and me. I thought perhaps Mom's blood sugar had dropped, so I went to get her an orange to eat.

Mom said she didn't want it. I told her I thought it would help her feel better. Mom threatened to call a cab to take her home if I cut the orange up and gave it to her.

In the back of mind, I was wondering what had prompted that extreme reaction, but I put the orange away immediately.

Mom was still angry when we left for dinner and stayed angry through the entire meal. It was miserable for my sister and me.

I kept trying to think of conversation topics that would lighten Mom's mood or not set her off more, but no matter what I brought up, it immediately disintegrated into anger from Mom.

Finally, I capitulated and we all ate - quickly - in silence.

My sister and I drove Mom back to her place and told her we loved her and we'd pick her up the next morning and bring her over and we'd do laundry and have lunch. Mom couldn't get away from us fast enough.

My sister and I talked about what had happened, but neither of us yet connected the dots because they were still too far apart to be a persistent pattern. We came to the conclusion that it was an anomaly brought on by low blood sugar.

We went to Mom's the next morning around 11 a.m. to pick up her. Mom wasn't in her room and her laundry wasn't in her room.

We walked around the building to see if we could find her.

Mom was sitting outside the dining room with a bunch of other residents waiting for the dining room to open for lunch. She didn't seem to recognize either my sister or me when we sat down on either side of her.

Eventually, Mom knew who we were, and when we asked her about laundry and lunch, she said she had her laundry going there and she was waiting for lunch.

We told her we'd go on then and be back later that afternoon to see her. My sister and I were pretty puzzled by this, but we still saw it as a weird aberration.

 However, after this, we decided that when we did go back, we'd ask Mom to go to dinner with us and if she said "no," we'd simply kiss her, tell her we loved her, and would go on without her.

Mom didn't want to go to dinner that evening – something was bothering her because she was not the least bit warm or fuzzy with either of us – and we went without her.

After that, however, things returned to normal and there wasn't any real evidence of a chronic problem that needed attention.

2009 was overall a good and calm year. Mom seemed to be doing well most of the time. She returned to more happy and chipper demeanor overall.

I began that year to handle Mom's medications, making sure they were filled on time, keeping up with changes, and making sure the dosages were in her weekly dispenser and taken as directed.

I kept a chart that Mom could refer to on her refrigerator so she knew exactly what she was taking and when.

The only hospitalization was in July when I took Mom in to see her P.A. and she was in full congestive heart failure and he called the hospital to have her admitted as soon I drove her over there.

I spent the entire time with her and we had good talks and very pleasant time together. Mom's cardiologist recommended a pacemaker and she had the implant done a couple of days later.

It was after that surgery that Mom got combative with my sister - who had come to town for the surgery - and me. We had done this enough to know it was time to tell Mom we loved her and leave.

We were at a restaurant that evening for dinner when my cell phone rang. I didn't recognize the number, so I didn't answer it. My sister said it might be the hospital, so I immediately called the number back.

The short version of the story was that Mom wanted to call the police to tell them the hospital was holding her against her will and she wanted to talk to me.

The nurse on Mom's wing called me to ask me to come and try to get Mom calmed down. In a series of missteps by the hospital in trying to get me and me to get them, the nurse had told Mom that she couldn't get me and that I must have been busy.

By the time I got through to the nurse, I told her that I would talk to Mom but I wouldn't come to the hospital because it would only make things worse. I recommended that she get Mom's doctor to prescribe a low-dosage anti-anxiety medication.

The phone that was in Mom's room wasn't working, so through after another convoluted series of steps, I finally had the nurse go to Mom's room, call me on that phone, and then let me talk to Mom. When she did and told Mom I was on the phone, Mom said "I don't want to talk to her. She's too busy to talk to me, so I'll just see her in the morning."

I hung up and just decided to let it go.

Mom was still irritated the next morning, but she lightened up as the day progressed.

We had a two-week follow-up appointment with Mom's P.A. after the pacemaker implant, so my sister suggested that I talk with him about adding a small-dose anti-anxiety medication for Mom, since a lot of this looked like anxiety.

I called the P.A.'s nurse, explained that I needed to talk to the P.A. before he saw Mom, so the anti-anxiety medication could be his idea and not mine. She told me she'd make it happen.

When Mom and I went back to the patient room, the P.A.'s nurse told me she'd come and get me to talk with the P.A. before he saw Mom.

She did and he agreed that Mom probably could benefit from anti-anxiety medication.

The nurse and I went back to the room where Mom was waiting and Mom was livid. She ordered both of us out of the room and said she wanted to talk to her doctor by herself.

The nurse was shocked. I wasn't, although I was surprised at how quickly Mom's disposition had gone south. We both warned the P.A. that a storm was well underway before he went in.

The P.A. was able to calm Mom down at least during the office visit, but she got angry at me again as soon as we got in the car. I filled the prescription for the anti-anxiety medication and made sure it was added to her weekly dispenser.

The next day everything was fine again and it remained that way until toward the end of the year.

In November, Mom began telling me that one of the residents was breaking into her room and taking her things. She told me she'd caught this residence twice in her room. In particular, there was some document - I don't remember what it was - that went missing and Mom accused this resident (they'd known each other several years and had always had this sort of "love/hate" relationship) to her face of stealing the document.

Not long after that, I found the document in Mom's papers and I showed it to Mom and told her she owed the lady she'd accused an apology. Whether that happened, I don't know.

However, the people coming in and out of Mom's room and snooping around in it became more frequent, but I assumed - wrongly - that it was cleaning or maintenance people that Mom just didn't recognize because the retirement community was having a high turnover in those two departments during that timeframe.

December brought another weird incident that I thought at the time was isolated. One of Mom's cousins died. The visitation was about fifty miles away, at night, which meant a drive of about one hundred miles round-trip. Mom wanted to go and she wanted to drive. I told Mom that I thought was a bad idea because she didn't need to be driving at night that distance by herself.

I told Mom if she wanted to go, I'd take her, and that I'd also go with her to the burial up in the cemetery where her mom's family was buried.

Mom got mad at me for telling her she shouldn't drive by herself and then hit me with a wall of tears and a rambling conversation about her family and her cousin and her aunt.

At some point, in the middle of all of that, however and to my relief, Mom decided not to go the visitation, but just to go to the burial.

We went to the burial which coincided with the start of an ice and snow storm, but Mom was calm and okay with just doing that by then.

Chapter 2: The Implosion

By the start of 2010, I began to realize that something pervasively wasn't right with Mom. As I'd do her medications each week, I noticed that Mom was missing dosages frequently and randomly.

Additionally, Mom forbade me from going to doctor's appointments with her.

In mid-January, Mom announced to me that the medications were killing her, that the pharmacy companies were stealing her money, and she'd found this diet that would solve all her medical problems and she'd talked to her P.A. and he'd agreed that she could stop all the medication and try the diet.

And Mom stopped all the medications that day. By then, I had decided to just let Mom do what she wanted to do unless she was putting herself or others in harm's way.

I picked my battles carefully and I knew money and stealing money had always been a fear and suspicion of Mom's, so I knew better than to argue or try to talk her out of the decision.

I also began to notice an increase in Mom's paranoia and suspicion - she'd had some of that all her life because of her early childhood - and also a weird mix of extreme clinginess with me alternating with a fierce pushing away.

I never knew which way that wind would be blowing each day when I went over to spend time with Mom, so inevitably both would always catch me off guard, for good or for bad.

One of the things that I also took note of early on that year was Mom telling me she was walking the halls a lot at night when she couldn't sleep. Even during the day, when I'd go over, we'd always take a long walk around the property. Often, we'd stop by the rocking chairs out back because Mom would get tired and we'd sit for an hour or so and rock and talk.

One morning in mid-March, Mom called me to tell me she had fallen backwards while walking outside. Mom said her head had hit the grass and she thought she was okay, but she asked me to come over.

I went over and Mom was okay, but clingy. I made sure that Mom was not hurt and stayed the rest of the day with her until she sent me home that evening, saying she was tired and was ready for bed. I made sure Mom was tucked in and left.

During the rest of March and April, when I wasn't working, I'd go over and spend several hours with Mom each day. Most of the time, she was glad for my company and we'd talk and spend time together.

Mom continued her routine of coming over to my place on Fridays to do our laundry and to help me clean the house and then I'd either take dinner over to her place or I'd bring her back to my house for dinner that evening.

Near the end of March, I was with Mom one day and she complained that her hearing aids weren't working well anymore.

Another thing that I had begun to notice was that, since the beginning of the year, Mom was spending more time in her apartment, and she would not put her hearing aids in until later in the day when she went out.

I was concerned about the isolation that suggested - which was not something Mom usually wanted - but I didn't say anything.

Often, by that point in time, when Mom did go out, there was a confrontation of some sort with the lady that Mom had accused of stealing from her at the end of 2009 (this lady sat out all day in the common areas, so it was impossible to avoid her).

Mom showed me an advertisement that she'd gotten somewhere for a new kind of hearing aids. She asked me what I thought about them and I suggested that we call and set up an appointment and check them out. Mom agreed and I made the appointment.

It was an expensive proposition for both hearing aids, but there was a 30-day money back guarantee, so Mom wanted to try them.

The technology was too complicated for Mom to try to figure out and two days later she told me they weren't working and she didn't want them.

I immediately took Mom with me back to the hearing aid place - she didn't want to go in - and told her I'd get the payment back, which I did. I showed Mom the refund receipt when I came back out to the car.

Mom apologized for not being able to use them and I told her there was nothing to apologize for.

I then suggested to Mom that we take her regular hearing aids to the audiology department at the local university, where she'd had them serviced before. Mom agreed to that and I made an appointment and we got them tuned up and refitted and Mom said they seemed to be working better.

In hindsight, I realize that we did this a lot over the next two years, and that the

TIA's, which by then were happening very frequently, were, because they affected her brain, affecting Mom's hearing.

In May, things started really getting dicey with Mom. Not all the time, but I could tell something big was starting to happen. Mom's mood swings escalated and her sudden anger-to-clinginess-back-to-anger toward me was becoming a fact of everyday life.

Late in the month, several things happened that made me consciously realize that something was seriously going wrong.

The first was that Mom was randomly trying to unsuccessfully pick fights with me and, whether I responded or didn't, no matter what I said, would then get absolutely furious with me, banishing me from her apartment after she'd spent her anger.

After I'd leave, she'd go and tell everyone else that I was just after her money, that I was stealing from her, that I wanted her out of the way (I didn't find out about this until July, although I suspected it in June). Nothing could have been further from the truth.

Mom's revocable trust was still in place with her as the trustee. While, because she asked me to help, I would sit down with Mom and make sure she paid her bills on time and would make sure she had printouts of her bank account balance, I had no access to any of her money.

I didn't want it, because I knew that money was also a sore spot with Mom and I didn't want that responsibility hanging over my head.

Around the same time, Mom was complaining more frequently about a boy and girl walking into her apartment every time she walked and just before she came back, they'd come out.

Once or twice she walked in while they were there and they were in the bathroom hanging towels.

Mom also, a couple of times, told me that Daddy had been to see her the night before. At the time, I thought maybe Mom was just having really vivid dreams that seemed real to her.

My way of dealing with this was just to listen to Mom and ask general questions to see if I could figure out what was going on.

Mom also started randomly driving some place on her own, without telling me, when we had planned to go together. That was probably the panic button that made me think more seriously about intervening and taking some action with Mom's P.A.

I remember the Friday before Memorial Day Mom showed up at my house around 8 a.m. and rang the doorbell instead of letting herself in (she had a key to my place).

I opened the door and said "Come on in!" and reached for Mom's arm to help her up take the step up into the house.

Mom grabbed my arm and hung on and I noticed she was shaking all over. I took her into the kitchen and got her seated and asked her if she'd eaten breakfast.

Mom seemed to be a slight daze, but answered me that she hadn't.

I thought maybe Mom's blood sugar had dropped and that was what was causing the trembling and the daze, so I fixed her a good breakfast and got her a cup of coffee and sat down with her while she ate.

Once Mom ate, the shaking stopped and she was herself again. I told Mom to sit tight and I'd go get her laundry and we'd get that done and she could rest in the recliner in the living room while it was washing and drying.

Mom agreed and I went to the car and there was no laundry.

After Mom had finished her coffee, I walked with her to the living room, sat her down in the recliner, and we spent the next two hours talking and discussing the day.

Then suddenly Mom popped out of the chair and wanted to go home. Mom seemed to be okay, but I suggested that I drive her home or at least that she'd let me follow her home. Mom insisted that she was fine and said she'd see me later, since I was bringing dinner over for us that night.

Mom left and I prayed. There is a four-way stop sign about an eighth of a mile from where I live, and that was the way Mom always went home, even though it's hairy for a good driver.

I had asked Mom to go the safer way, but she was used to her way, so she wouldn't change.

About thirty minutes after Mom left, my sister called and I told her what had happened.

My sister was very upset about me letting Mom drive herself home and asked me if she'd gotten home okay. I couldn't think of anything else to say except, "well, if Mom crashed, I'm close enough to hear it, and it's been quiet, so she made it home okay."

Mom was okay later in the day when I went over with dinner, so I thought maybe the morning incident really was a blood sugar issue.

That following Monday, I took Mom out driving for the day. We went to the cemetery where Mom's mother and her mother's family are buried. After that, we went down to the cemetery where her father, her father's family, and my dad are buried.

After we left the second cemetery, there was one new, odd thing that happened.

Mom said she wanted to go see her grandpa's house. I knew which house Mom meant, even though I'd never heard her until that day refer to it as "Grandpa's house."

The house Mom was referring to had, until that time, been her Aunt Tilda's house. It was close to the paternal cemetery, but I had never heard Mom refer to it as her grandpa's house until then.

I took Mom there and as we drove by and saw what the remaining family who owned the house had done with it (it was in a serious state of decay and junk had been piled up on the porch and around it), Mom's mood suddenly darkened and she began to try to start an argument with me.

One thing I did learn quickly was not to take Mom's bait. I'd get quiet, which also made her angry, but at least I wasn't giving her any of my words to twist and throw back at me in a configuration that I didn't even recognize.

I took Mom to lunch, but things deteriorated even further, so instead of taking her back to my house afterwards, I dropped her off at her place.

I kept thinking there must be something I was doing wrong or that I was saying that was setting Mom off and I really undertook a deep self-appraisal to fix the problems I could see in myself that could be contributing to what was going on with Mom.

And that's a good lesson and thing that came out of all of this. I'm not the same person I was going into it and that's a good thing. I'm still not where I want or need to be, but I've made progress and continue to pursue progress, so that was a positive outcome for me.

I had learned by this time that time and space were the only chance Mom and I had to "start over" each day on a better footing.

I had also learned that trying to stay and "fix" what was broken only made it worse and escalated it into a full-blown war as far as Mom was concerned.

Once Mom was in that mode, she could get startling vicious and nasty and would rip me to shreds six ways from Sunday, which was always crushingly devastating for me, although Mom never seemed to remember it happening after the fact.

That quote about everything being fair in love and war is not true.

The week after that was relatively quiet, but then Mom took off alone in the car on that Saturday when we were supposed to be going together in my car, with me driving. Mom didn't tell me what she was doing. Mom just did it.

This was the breaking point for me with Mom driving. I called my sister, told her what had happened, and she agreed with me that Mom needed to stop driving.

We also both agreed that her P.A. had to be the one to tell Mom, because if we did it, she'd go on full-tilt rampage against us both. My sister said she'd come up the next day and we'd work to get an appointment with the P.A. as early in the week as possible.

I got to my destination and didn't see Mom's car, but someone checked and Mom was there.

By now, I knew I was dealing with dementia of some sort, and I knew I had to take immediate action for Mom's safety and protection without getting her upset and angry at me.

Afterwards, I found Mom's car and she was standing by it. I could tell Mom was angry.

Mom told me that she'd stopped to get gas and she'd broken the passenger door mirror, but she didn't know how it got broken. It was shattered, so I can only imagine that Mom hit something at the gas station.

I told Mom that we'd take the back way home and I'd follow her to her place to make sure she got home okay.

It was a heart-pounding drive for me. Mom was all over the road and I spent the entire trip praying that she wouldn't hit somebody or drift over into oncoming traffic. We got to Mom's place safely, but my decision was made.

I walked in with Mom to her apartment and seeing that she was still angry and wanted to get into it with me, I kissed her goodbye, told her I loved her (I always did these two things no matter how badly things were going between us until she took her last breath), and that I'd see her the next morning.

I probably waited a little too long to take action, but I think, given the same situation again, I'd do the same thing. Mom was always fiercely independent and I was determined to let her have as much independence as she was able as long as she lived.

I had watched other people care for loved ones with some form of dementia and I watched those loved ones' internal lights fade quickly as everything early on in the diseases was taken away from them and out of their control.

I was determined - and because I was Mom's medical POA - not to do that to Mom. I took a lot of heat from my sister who was most involved for doing this and she always accused me of not doing something sooner for my own selfish reasons.

As I took stock of those accusations, I realize that early on in this process with Mom, there was some reluctance on my part to take all that responsibility on myself, but it was not selfishness.

Part of it was simply me. I have never made many promises or commitments in my life, because I realized the seriousness of doing that and the responsibility it put on me to keep them. That responsibility, once encumbered, was not negotiable.

I knew and know myself well enough to know that I tend to be a runner. In most areas of my life, I've kept connections loose and distant and made sure that I had plenty of escape routes if things got too intense, too heavy, and so much so that the runner in me kicked in and I needed to, had to, was compelled to run away.

I will never be able to explain that in tangible terms, in words that would make sense to anyone else. But it was a truth that I knew - and know - about me.

So at each step of the process with Mom, I had to review my promise to Dad and to Mom to take care of Mom.

I had to make sure I was ready to do whatever it took to keep that promise.

I wasn't always ready when Mom needed me to be, but eventually, I always kept those promises. I regret my own shortcomings in not always being ready at the same time Mom really needed me to be.

Another reason that entered my thought processes was that I couldn't bear the thought of seeing Mom simply give up on life too soon as I had seen those people give up and I was determined not to limit Mom's freedom any more than was absolutely necessary because I knew it would kill her spirit.

I'm enough like Mom in that way to understand what being totally dependent on someone else would do to me, and I was not willing to do that to her.

My sister and I were able to meet with P.A. early Tuesday morning. Since Mom had forbidden me since the beginning of the year to go to doctor's appointments, I simply had to depend on what Mom told me was the result of those appointments was what was going on.

I had ten pages in a list of things that pointed to some form of dementia that I took in with me. Mom's P.A. told us that he had been noticing the changes and had given her, at her last appointment, the week before, the simple cognitive test for dementia and Mom and she'd failed it completely.

I told him that I'd noticed speech issues (using the wrong words for things) with Mom and he said that he believed she had a mild form of vascular dementia (he'd ordered a CT scan for Wednesday and was to see Mom on Thursday with the results).

I have emails from Mom during that time period, as well as typed and hand-written documents, and it's clear just how scrambled her brain was.

Mom was not thinking in full sentences and her thought processes were merging events of the distant past with the present in an inaccurate perception of what was actually going on.

There are many documents where Mom started typing and there are just a few random words (the same words, so it was something that was on her mind) because Mom couldn't complete the thought.

I found a document Mom started where she had typed that Daddy died in December 1998 (which was a biggie for me, because he died October 15, 1998 and it was a date Mom had etched in her memory because I saw it time and again in writing she'd done after his death).

Mom's handwritten documents follow the same few random words pattern, and the handwriting is illegible (Mom always had beautiful cursive writing, while Daddy's handwriting identified him as a doctor because it was often hard to read) and scrawled down the page.

We all agreed that Mom needed to stop driving and the P.A. said that he wanted us to come with Mom on Thursday for the appointment and he'd tell her while we were there and he'd let all know what the results of the CT scan were.

My sister and I spent the next day with Mom until she left for the CT exam. Mom had not told me about it, but had gotten the retirement community's transportation people to give her a ride there and back. Even as she was leaving, she didn't tell us anything except that she was going for a doctor's appointment.

When Mom got back, she said she thought had an appointment with her P.A. that week too, but she couldn't remember. She asked if I would call and check for her.

I did and told Mom that Deb and I would take her on Thursday and then take her to lunch. We told Mom that we wanted to make sure we knew what was going on so we could help her.

Amazingly, Mom agreed. So, the next morning we all went to the P.A. The CT scan showed small vessel ischemia (the result of a lifetime of TIA's) all over her brain. The layman's version is that each TIA had deprived a small section of her brain of oxygen and that area of the brain had died (the brain is the one organ in the body that does not regenerate itself, so when cells or tissue die, they are dead for good).

Mom had had so many of these TIA's that there were clusters of these dead "zones" that were affecting the ability of her brain to communicate and function the way it was supposed to. The P.A.

referred to it as multi-infarct dementia, but said he believed it was mild and might be managed with some vitamin supplements.

He also gave me the number of a geriatric psychiatrist to contact and get an appointment for Mom with (I did that as soon as I got home, but the appointment was not until early August).

The P.A. then told Mom that she had asked him to tell her when she needed to stop driving, so they were at that point and she couldn't drive anymore.

Mom protested a little, but finally accepted what he said. I assured Mom, as did her P.A., that I was her on-call ride anytime she needed or wanted to go somewhere, no questions asked, so she'd never be without transportation.

Mom didn't seem upset when we left. We went to lunch and then went to pick up the vitamin supplements her P.A. had recommended and then went back to Mom's place.

And all hell broke loose as soon as my sister and I started gathering up all the car keys. Mom railed and ranted at us that we weren't taking her keys and no one was taking her car and she ordered us to leave. We'd managed to get all the keys we could find, so we left.

Mom never drove again after that and by the next day she had calmed down about it.

I began spending more time with Mom to make sure she could go wherever she wanted to go and do whatever she wanted or needed to do.

I quickly became aware of what Mom must have been doing on a daily basis those few months prior to being told she shouldn't be driving anymore.

One of those things was going to the bank every couple of days to check on her account balances. I'd sit in the car while Mom would go in and she'd be in there for quite a while and then come back out to the car with a little Post-It note with her balances handwritten on it. Mom would quickly put it in her purse so I wouldn't see it.

The other thing Mom did was make almost daily mini-trips to the grocery store and to the drugstore. She'd pick up two or three items each visit. I was somewhat aware of this because I was helping Mom keep her checkbook balanced and up-to-date, but I didn't realize this was almost a daily ritual.

Because I was with Mom most of the time by then, I really began to see just how much confusion, paranoia, and suspicion had begun to take root in her thinking.

Mom's moods were wildly vacillating from sudden rage to terrible fear to heart-breaking apologies and tears. Any one of those could appear and disappear suddenly.

In retrospect, I can only imagine how scary this must have been for Mom.

Combined with Mom's hearing loss, which sometimes isolated her in group situations because she couldn't make out conversations - although she was an excellent lip-reader - with all the voices coming at her simultaneously ending up being nothing but an incomprehensible and confusing jumble of sound, this was probably terrifying to her.

In addition, because suspicion and paranoia were everpresent components, Mom must have believed that there was no human - including me - that she could trust.

I know Mom never lost her faith or trust in God and in Jesus Christ. I suspect during that time, they were the only two beings in the universe Mom believed she could depend on.

The week after Mom stopped driving, a friend of mine came to town for a couple of days en route to her home.

Mom had known my friend for a long time and considered her to be another daughter.

My friend and I made plans to go out with Mom for the first day and we began a pleasant trip to the cemeteries where Mom wanted to go.

The morning part of the drive was fine, but as we headed out to the other cemetery, Mom's mood began to change.

I've always believed I somehow precipitated this particular change because of a driver who got on my bumper and wouldn't back off as I turned down the narrow country road that led out to the second cemetery. I expressed my concern out loud and there must have been enough fear in my voice that Mom picked up on it and immediately started getting agitated and anxious.

I tried to lose the driver by turning down the road that led to the house that Mom, since our Memorial Day drive out there, was now calling "Grandpa's house." The driver turned with me and stayed right on my bumper. I got anxious because that shouldn't have happened and I was now concerned that I was dealing with a psycho driver who could harm all of us.

In another attempt to lose the driver, I turned into the driveway of "Grandpa's house." My heart started pounding with fear when the driver turned in behind me and stopped the car. By now, Mom's agitation was full-blown and she wanted to get out of the car and confront the driver.

I kept the car running while I could assess how to safely get out of the situation. The doors were locked and the windows were rolled up, so Mom was not able to get out of the car. Mom was yelling and screaming at me to let her out as she was trying to open the door. Both my friend and I told Mom that it wasn't a good idea and it could be dangerous.

Mom was in a full rage by then and began flinging herself against the door to try to get it open. Afraid that Mom was going to hurt herself, I turned off the car, and as soon as the door unlocked, she jumped out and almost ran toward the other driver to get in her face and confront her. I was out of the car right behind Mom trying to figure out what I was going to do if this whole thing went south.

Mom ranted and raved at the other driver about the condition of "Grandpa's house" and demanded to talk to "Jimmy" about it. The driver stayed calm - it ended up that she worked for some of Mom's cousins who now owned the house - and called one of the cousins who said he'd be down to talk to Mom shortly.

Mom didn't wait. She got back in the car and demanded to leave. As I drove away, I was pretty shaken. I thought about what Mom had said to the driver and wondered who "Jimmy" was.

A few miles down the road, I realized that Jimmy was one of Mom's favorite cousins who had died a few days short of his seventeenth birthday in a tractor accident on the farm many years before.

I had no idea where Mom was in time and I understood that she didn't either. Mom had calmed down considerably and wanted to take us to lunch, so we went to lunch. After lunch, we went back to Mom's place and spent several pleasant hours together. It was as if the earlier events were just a figment of my imagination.

This was the aspect that I had the hardest time dealing with. I don't switch gears quickly or easily so the sudden twists and turns would upend me and it seemed as if I was off balance all the time and couldn't find something steady and reliable to hold on to through all the storms and upheavals.

I also had a very hard time comprehending and accepting that Mom could go from one extreme to another without knowing, remembering, or having any lingering effects.

I kept trying to apply logic, reason, and rationality to something that was illogical, unreasonable, and irrational and that created a lot of mental and psychological pain for me.

It is still painful for me now when I think about it because I couldn't, I can't, and I will never be able to make any of it make sense.

That's one of the sadder things about dementias. My only consolation is that it was - and is - a longer duration for me, time-wise, than it was for Mom, and Mom really had no long-term memories of any of that time. That's a blessing, in my opinion.

The next morning I took my friend to the airport and then went over to see Mom. Mom wasn't in her apartment when I got there, so I looked around and found her sitting at a table on the covered patio out back. I smiled as I opened the door to the patio, but as soon as Mom's eyes met mine, I knew she was in a dark place.

Even when I was a kid, Mom always had a look that let me know she was angry and I was in trouble.

Mom never lost that look.

Even after I grew up, that look could stop me dead in my tracks and I'd revert internally to that little kid wondering what in the world I'd done this time to rock Mom's world. But as dementia took hold, I saw this look more and more frequently.

In hindsight, I realize that this was the turning point for Mom in what turned out to be a three-week rollercoaster ride that resulted in Mom being involuntarily committed in early July, after she made a 3 a.m. ranting and raving call to 911 and was transported to the hospital with the home safe she kept in her apartment, to a psychiatric geriatric hospital.

I was notified early that Sunday morning and told what to bring to the geriatric psychiatric hospital when I got there to change it to a voluntary commitment by me.

I had already, a couple of weeks earlier, talked with the attorney who had drawn up Mom's revocable trust and let him know what was going on and that Mom was mentally not competent to make any changes to it (Mom never tried and it never came up in a conversation, but I knew he needed a heads up).

I went to Mom's apartment and straightened up, finding a notebook that Mom had accused me of stealing stuck in the one place I had not looked - behind her dresser - when I searched for it a few days before as she was threatening to call the police and have me arrested, checked for bills that needed to be paid and paid them, and packed a bag for her.

I was sort of in a daze. I had not slept much or well the week before and had been awake most of the night before just trying to figure out - and praying for help - what to do about Mom.

I was having a hard time squaring the "mild vascular dementia" that Mom's P.A. had diagnosed a month earlier with the precipitous steep and rapid decline I'd seen since then.

Of all the people I'd seen with dementias, the progress was slower and more subtle over time with small downturns along the way. What I had seen with Mom was something completely different and I didn't know what that meant for her and me going forward.

Mom and I had, at her suggestion, taken a tour of a memory-care facility (external doors were locked to ensure that residents didn't get out and wander around and get hurt or killed - I had found out, after the fact, that Mom had done this one night in late June and ended up at the local hospital for the night) that was run by the same company that owned the independent living community, so I figured that was going to be the next step if and until Mom was stabilized.

I didn't even know if Mom could be stabilized, but I knew in Mom's untreated condition, it was impossible for me to keep her safe, secure, and happy. That made me sad because there was nothing I could do to fix things for her. Believe me, if I could have, I would have.

And there wasn't a day that passed that I wouldn't have gladly gone through everything Mom was going through so she wouldn't have to.

No matter how angry and vicious and nasty Mom got toward me, I loved her unconditionally and I would have traded places with her in a heartbeat because I would have rather hurt than to see Mom hurt.

I don't know if Mom ever really understood that, but there wasn't a day that passed by until the end of her life that I didn't hold her hands, look in her eyes, and tell her that.

I went to the geriatric psychiatric hospital early that afternoon and I was not prepared for what I walked into.

It was jarring and heartbreaking at the same time.

If I'd had to describe it in one word, "chaos" would have been the word.

There was screaming and mumbling and crying all around. Elderly folks were shuffling around the check-in desk and sitting in wheelchairs behind me and down the hall, all in their own worlds and conversations. The smell of human waste from bladder and bowel incontinence was overpowering.

And inside I was screaming and crying that my mama didn't belong here like this, with these crazy people, and my heart was ripping in two because I realized logically this was the right next step and this hospital was the only option for Mom (the other mental health hospital would not take elderly patients) to get stabilized, if possible, and back to some of kind of decent life, but I hated it for her.

The staff and the facility reminded me of all the worst descriptions I've read and seen about mental hospitals. There seemed to be an indifference and lack of real care and concern about the patients. There seemed to be a lack of concern and care about hygiene and cleanliness in general. It seemed that the inmates were running the asylum.

Fighting all my internal protests, I signed the voluntary commitment for Mom. While I was doing the paperwork, Mom was brought up in a wheelchair and she went right by me without recognizing me. I fought back tears - for all that Mom had already lost and all the unknowns going forward (I wasn't sure Mom was ever going to be "back" in any way that she'd know me) - as I completed her admission and handed over her packed bag.

Visiting hours were very limited – and required being buzzed in after identification – each day, but I was determined to go daily the two times a day I could see Mom, as well call each morning and evening to check on how Mom had done during the day and then during the night.

I left and cried all the way home. Once I got home, I realized I needed to stop crying and get to work on taking care of Mom and handling everything that needed to be handled.

I'd called my sisters and niece earlier that day to tell them what was going on, and after I got the hospital information, I emailed them contact information and times.

The next two weeks were a whirlwind of stuff that I needed to get done yesterday. I went to the bank on Monday and started the process of making sure I had the access to take care of Mom's financial matters (I would need to letter from the psychiatrist at the hospital to state that Mom was no longer competent to handle her affairs for the bank) and started the process of getting Mom moved out of the independent living community to the memory-care community.

While I was visiting Mom during the first noon visit – Mom knew me, but she was anxious and wasn't really sure where she was, so she was distracted by that – the social worker asked me to meet with her on my way out.

The social worker was not very warm and fuzzy, like the rest of the staff there. The conversation was short and abrupt as she gave me my marching orders that I needed to complete by the time Mom was released in two weeks.

One thing the social worker said to me that really made me angry was that I needed to forget about emotions – I had not showed any emotion, so I'm not where this came from – and buck up and get everything done. I know social workers get burned out after years on the job, but I was not expecting the coldness and rudeness she spoke with.

I told the social worker that I needed a letter from the psychiatrist to be able to execute the trust and have the legal authority to take care of Mom's affairs and she made an appointment for me to meet with him the next morning.

I spent the rest of that afternoon before I went back for the evening visit making a to-do list for the next two weeks. My sister and niece both called and said they'd be in the following week to help getting Mom packed up and moved.

I met with the psychiatrist the next morning where he gave me the letter for the legal authority I needed for handling Mom's affairs and he told me that Mom had mid-to-late-stage vascular dementia and Alzheimer's Disease.

I was simultaneously surprised and not surprised by this diagnosis. I was surprised because a month earlier, Mom's P.A. had said she had mild vascular dementia and there was no mention of Alzheimer's Disease. I was not surprised because it explained everything I'd been seeing and experiencing with Mom.

I asked if it could be treated and managed. The psychiatrist said that there were anti-psychotic medications that could control the hallucinations and delusions, mood stabilizers that could help keep Mom's brain chemistry more stable, a stronger form of anti-anxiety medication, and cognitive enhancement medications that could help counteract some of the dementia and Alzheimer's symptoms.

He said the next week or so would be spent getting the right dosages of each to stabilize Mom so she could be released. I asked him if he'd be willing to provide a final list and dosage for the new drugs. He said he would.

I had three hours before my noon visit with Mom so I went and made copies of the psychiatrist letter and gave a copy to the bank to ensure that I had access to Mom's bank accounts to pay her bills and stopped by her P.A.'s office to let him know what was going on, to get the current list of prescriptions he had prescribed for Mom that she wasn't taking, and to get a handicap placard signed by him for my car since I'd been using Mom's placard up until that point, but I knew I was going to be selling her car and putting whatever I got for it into her savings account.

I didn't expect to see Mom's P.A. when I stopped by. I left a message with the front desk and they asked me to wait while they called his nurse. A few minutes later, his nurse came up and said that Mom's P.A. wanted to see me.

I don't think he expected Mom's diagnosis either and I think it really shook him up that that's where she was.

But the thing that surprised me most was that as I was talking about Mom he stopped me and asked "how are you doing?" I started talking about Mom again and he stopped me again and asked me the same question.

I am sure I said I was okay, but that is my standard response no matter what's going on. But then he asked me if I was sleeping. I can only imagine that the fatigue and stress that I was oblivious to was staring him in the face.

He was very kind and gentle and he suggested - and gave me samples of - a non-narcotic sleep medicine and a very mild anti-anxiety medication and urged me to take them temporarily (and I didn't, of course, except for the anti-anxiety medication on two occasions when the stress got so bad I thought I was going to break) for the next two weeks.

He said something to me that I hope that I never forget: "you are one the strongest people I know and this doesn't mean you're weak, but when the strongest people finally break under the weight of everything they're trying to handle, they fall and crash hard and it can be very difficult to get back up."

He told me to call him if I needed anything and he'd work me in. Of all the medical professionals I worked with that first week of Mom's hospitalization, his kindness and concern, not just for Mom, but for me as well, was in stark contrast to basic indifference and lack of concern from the rest in that field.

That P.A. will always have a soft spot in my heart, even though near the end of Mom's life when I couldn't get him to understand that Mom was dying and I needed his acceptance and cooperation to make sure that it was as easy, comfortable, and peaceful for her as possible and I had to change to partner with a doctor in the same group who'd been also heavily involved in Mom's care and was on the same page with me, because of his gentleness and tenderness.

As I was to learn, this care and concern was both his greatest strength and his greatest weakness, but I was grateful for it when I needed it.

My days the rest of that week were filled with my twice-a-day visits to Mom (sometimes Mom was okay and sometimes she wasn't) and getting the move and all the legal and financial things taken care of so that I could take care of Mom.

By the time Mom was released on the Friday of the second week (the director of nursing who evaluated her made sure I got a list of all the medications Mom was released with), my family who had come to town to help me with the packing, the moving, and making Mom's new apartment look like home and I were holding our breath to see how Mom was and it was going to go.

My sister and I had seen Mom still quite angry and paranoid and delusional just a few days earlier on a visit, so I wasn't sure those symptoms could be dealt with that quickly. I remember that visit with Mom because she reminded me of the Looney Toons character Taz because of the way she would spin in a counter-clockwise vortex when she got out of control (the term off-kilter comes to mind) and we both had to catch her because the spinning left her off balance.

I'd never seen Mom do that before, but from that day until she died, that same elaborate motion was how Mom would turn around and I think most of her falls -

fortunately, there were no broken bones and no earth-shattering damage to her, although watching a few of them because she was just out of my reach and I couldn't get there fast enough to catch her, I know she had to have a contingency of angels around her breaking the falls - were a result of that spinning motion.

I don't know what caused it. And I've never seen another person suffering with dementia do it, even those with the additional diagnosis of Lewy Body dementia, which I saw sporadic symptoms of after Mom's release from the hospital, but which was full-blown by the end of 2011.

That's one of the few unanswered questions I have left, and I've accepted that I'll never know the reason behind it.

Chapter 3: After the Implosion

While we all waited nervously at Mom's new place for her arrival by ambulance, hoping that Mom would like what we'd done with it and that she'd transition well, the director of nursing came in to talk with us and tell us that Mom was in good spirits when she saw her earlier that morning and she thought the psychiatrist had gotten her on the right medication regimen. She was very reassuring that it was going to be okay.

And she was right, much to my surprise. Mom came in smiling, recognizing all of us, and hugging us and telling us she loved us. Mom loved her new apartment and she was genuinely glad we were there with her.

I confess that my anxiety levels that it wouldn't last didn't go down for a few months until I saw continual evidence that the medications were working and that Mom was happier and more calm - she was still Mom in all her spunkiness and humor, which had also been one of the concerns that I had with her being medicated - and all the worries, paranoia and suspicion was gone. Mom never asked me about her finances, how things were paid for, or worried about it, which was a tremendous relief to me.

However, I had no idea what I had undertaken when I took over managing all the details of Mom's life. I don't know how even healthy elderly people, without help and advocacy from their families, handle all the things that are involved with doctors, Medicare, pharmaceutical companies, medication, and hospitalizations. It is a tremendous amount of work of and by itself.

I began, after Mom's hospitalization, a folder with all Mom's legal and medical paperwork, including her DNR and all the powers of attorney paperwork, that I took everywhere with me when Mom and I were together. I also kept an updated list of her current medications in there as well.

I had taken Mom's purse home with me the day she was hospitalized and bought a wallet that just had her driver's license, her credit card (I'd already, over the previous years because she kept losing her wallet and I'd have to cancel all the credit cards, pared her credit cards down to just one), her pacemaker card, and her Medicare and Part B insurance cards. I kept that wallet in the backpack with her pertinent information folder.

It made things so much easier for me because I made appointments, dealt with hospital and doctors' offices check-ins and check-outs, and, except for the subsequent visits with the psychiatrist, was the one who helped Mom explain things to the medical professionals and bring any current issues to their attention. I highly recommend this method of having everything you need in one place when you need it.

I wasn't sure at first how being without a purse was going to sit with Mom. Mom's purse was like another appendage for her and I thought she would want a purse with her. But she didn't. Mom never looked for it, asked me about it, or ever carried one with her again.

I had planned, if Mom had wanted one, to give her a purse filled with tissues, a pen, a little notebook, and mints that would be no big deal if she lost it or left it somewhere.

But, to my surprise, Mom had forgotten that she'd ever carried a purse and even seeing other ladies with purses didn't trigger the memory for her.

The first order of business after Mom was released was getting her a replacement social security card. I knew Mom had one somewhere because I'd seen it, but I was not able to find it in any of her belonging after she went into the hospital.

I needed the social security card to get a veteran's pension for Mom for assisted living from the VA because Dad served during the Korean War.

If one or both of your parents served during a period of war, they or their spouses are eligible for this monthly benefit, which helps offset some of the cost of assisted living. You'll need the following documentation to apply:

- The veteran's discharge form (DD-214)
- Both parents' social security cards (if the spouse is the widow or widower of a veteran)
- A copy of their marriage certificate
- An itemized list of monthly income and expenses (be sure to include supplemental insurance payments, medication expenses, including the Medicare "donut hole" increases for patented drugs, life insurance payments, etc.)

You can apply online, but be aware that if you do not have the DD-214, although you can request a copy of it online, that there was a fire in 1973 at the main army and air force records archive in St. Louis, MO and Army records from 1912 to 1961 and Air Force records from 1947 to 1964 were destroyed.

If the veteran is in one of those two branches of service during those time frames, there is another option, although it may be a long shot, for possibly obtaining a copy of the DD-214 by contacting his or her employer (if he or she retired recently) because the employers usually have a copy of this as part of the hiring paperwork for veteran personnel.

If you do not get a timely approval on the benefit, take a trip to your local VA office. It's worth the wait because the face-to-face meeting, which I ended up having to do, gets immediate results and the benefit starts shortly thereafter and continues until your loved one dies.

I also recommend setting up a monthly budget of your loved one's income and expenses (I used an Excel spreadsheet and updated it as expenses or payments increased or decreased and kept it with the check register so I could put in the automatic debits and credits at the beginning of each month so I had an accurate checking account balance at all times), as well as a 12-month folder system of receipts and deposits so if you need them, you have them.

This is especially important in the case where one of the children is the POA, but your loved ones have a dispersion will that leaves a portion of what's left (if anything, because all of this gets very expensive) to all their children so that you can give the rest of the inheritors an accurate accounting of how your loved ones' money was spent and what for.

It's a shame that that's often what the kids fight over when the parents are gone, and that is precisely why Mom set up the revocable trust with her as the primary trustee and me as the secondary trustee. Mom knew I was her primary caretaker and had been since Dad's death and would be until she died.

Mom told me she didn't want me to have to deal with any battles over an inheritance (and there was not one, but I'd always told her that any money she had was for her and not me or any of us and it would be used to take care of her and that's what happened).

Mom settled in beautifully at the assisted living community and got active and I made sure she got any therapy she needed to improve cognitively, physically, and any other way that would improve her quality of life. I made sure I was there every day, often at different times of the day, for several hours. I knew all the staff and they all knew me.

That is very important for caregivers to do. You need to be a constant presence. It is the only way to ensure that everyone is living up to the agreement the community made to you and your loved one when you entered a contract with them.

I knew Mom's stay at this community would be only until she needed my full-time care and then she'd be coming home with me.

The only reasons I didn't bring Mom home with me after the hospitalization was because I wasn't sure how or if the medication was going to work and I didn't want for Mom to be alone and not around people her own age and have as much human interaction as she needed and wanted, because I knew that was vital to her happiness and her thriving.

Being an end-spectrum introvert myself, I am perfectly content - and often need this to recharge - to unplug as soon as I'm able from all human contact. I do fine with business human interaction, but by the end of the work day, I'm done.

It's nothing against anyone. I just reach my saturation level and I need to be alone. I don't socialize much and, if I do, because I know that's expected, even though I tend to avoid it at all cost because of the energy drain, it's only for short periods of time because that's all I can take.

I'm very protective of any "free" time because I need that to recharge and get mentally prepared for the next block of "non-free" time.

I can't be around people all the time without crashing and burning and actually becoming next to impossible to be around anyway.

Mom, though, was different and I knew she thrived on being around other people - Mom was always wanted to help others and I saw her doing that with some of the other residents as soon as she got settled in the memory-care facility - so I knew she needed a place where she had a lot of people her own age around.

One of the things I did - and recommend - is to build good relationships with the nursing staff (especially the director of nursing) and with the CNAs. You'll know in a very short period of time who will watch out for your loved ones and make sure problems get addressed and resolved right away and who, quite frankly, is just there for a paycheck. I built some great relationships there and there are several nurses and CNAs that I still count among my friends.

This is critical because it affects the quality of care your loved one will receive. Don't complain all the time and decide what are important issues to pursue and what are minor ones to let slide. Work with them as partners and show them respect and gratitude and they will respond in the most amazing ways.

Also be sure to deal directly with the nursing staff on all medication changes or additions and special dietary needs or restrictions.

One of the on-going – and it was really the only complaint I had overall with this community – was that although Mom's P.A. had prescribed a low-fat, heart-healthy diet for Mom since her blood pressure and congestive heart failure issues were becoming problematic, the diet was not adhered to by all the staff.

I actually began taking in sugar-free and low-desserts for the kitchen to include with Mom's meals so that she could have dessert with everyone else. We never got it completely right, but at least I was able to control it to some degree.

Mom thrived there for a little over a year, but then had a serious fall in September of 2011. It happened at night and it was not handled correctly by the CNA. Fortunately, although it was painful for

Mom, she suffered only a severely sprained ankle, but I had already started realizing that Mom needed to come home and live with me because her need for care was increasing. I spent the next two weeks living there with Mom so that her ankle could heal and so I'd be there to help her shower, get up at night and go to the bathroom, and be there to assist her 24/7.

In early October, I went to see Mom on my daily visit, and I noticed she was having an extremely hard time breathing. I told Mom I thought we needed to get her into the doctor to get it checked out. I made an appointment that morning and Mom's P.A. said it could either be pneumonia or the beginning of congestive heart failure, but he would treat it as pneumonia with an antibiotic and breathing treatments to see if that cleared it up.

A week or so later, as I often did, I brought Mom home to spend some time with me away from the community. Mom was happy to be home with me, but I noticed how easily she got fatigued and I also noticed over the next couple of days how difficult breathing was for her.

After a night of listening to Mom's ragged breath while sleeping, when Mom woke up that morning, I told her we were going to get dressed and go to the hospital because her breathing didn't sound good. Mom agreed.

Mom was in full congestive heart failure and was admitted to pull all the excess fluid off her heart and out of her lungs. She stayed for five days. When Mom was discharged I brought her back home with me and Mom told me she wanted to stay with me and not go back. I asked Mom if she wanted to live with me, and she said, "yes."

I knew it was time and so we agreed that Mom would live with me from then on. We got Mom packed up and moved in and I turned the living room, where I had a couch that unfolded into a queen size bed and where we slept until a couple of months before Mom died when the recliner was more comfortable for her (I slept on the couch and she slept in the chair) and then the last few days Mom was alive we got a hospital bed moved in there for her, into Mom's bedroom.

The downstairs of the house became our living area since Mom wasn't able to climb the stairs to the bedrooms and full bath up there.

I wasn't sure how I was going to work it all out, but I got creative and found ways to give Mom baths and wash her hair without a shower, which was my biggest concern.

There was another hospitalization shortly after Mom came to stay with me - a temporary relapse into the pre-dementia-medication behavior - and it was determined that the primary issue was that Mom's oxygen saturation levels were very low, so we got oxygen for her to use all the time.

Mom and I settled into a routine of putting puzzles together, walking as she could tolerate it (we had home health and physical therapy until hospice took over just before she died), reading, and other activities to keep her mind as active as possible. I made sure that, for as long as Mom was able, we got out of the house as often as possible, if nothing more than to drive around for a while, and we went grocery shopping, to the mall to walk, to the bookstores in town, to the library, and occasionally out to lunch or to dinner.

I will always remember that period of time fondly and I treasure the fact that I was able to be with Mom, take care of her, and be right beside her all the way to the last breath.

Mom did well physically until January 2012. Although she'd been hospitalized just after Thanksgiving with tardive dyskinesia, which was a delayed reaction to SeroquelXR (the anti-psychotic drug she'd been taking since July 2010), and that had been discontinued and replaced with a mood stabilizer that wouldn't stop the hallucinations and the delusions, but would make sure they didn't scare Mom, she was relatively happy and alert most of the time and doing pretty well, all things considered.

I remember distinctly the first night in December of 2011, a couple of weeks after Mom had stopped the Seroquel RX, when she asked me while we were eating dinner at the kitchen table if my mom and dad were still alive. Then she asked where I was going to college and what I was majoring in.

In spite of this completely catching me off guard, I answered Mom's questions with the actual facts of my life. And that made Mom happy. But I realized that Mom didn't know who I was.

These episodes of Mom not recognizing me started sporadically, but they were quickly increasing in frequency. Mom wasn't afraid of me, but she didn't always know me. When Mom would ask me who my mother was and I'd point to her, she'd get a quizzical look on her face and ask "I'm your mother?" I'd nod and Mom would accept it.

These instances of Mom not knowing who I was didn't last long until near the end of her life when, except for the day of complete alertness before and the morning of the day she started her death sleep, she didn't know who I was for a little over a week.

The first week of January, though, Mom had no energy. She wasn't sick, but she stayed in bed for two days and slept almost continually. Mom was very clingy and I stayed close by and we had some heartbreaking talks and we had some good talks, but I wasn't sure she wasn't dying then.

Mom recovered and seemed to get a little stronger physically, but I started noticing the symptoms that I was able to identify as Lewy Body dementia come on her full-tilt. I think the SeroquelXR had calmed these symptoms down and once she was off of that medication, they came back to the surface.

When the symptoms started, they surprised me. I'd be in the kitchen working on something after Mom went to bed and she'd start talking. Most of it was hard to understand, but I'd go in to see if Mom needed me, and she was asleep talking, and moving her hands in the air in very animated conversations with someone. Mom would nod or shake her head and verbally agree or disagree, all while sleeping. It would go on most of the night and lasted until a week or so before she died.

Sometimes, if Mom was really restless, I'd hold her hand throughout the night and that would calm her down some.

There were a lot tender moments and hugs that I remember during this time and I'm grateful for that. I'm also grateful that Mom was able to communicate with me up until the very end. Although Mom's comprehension waxed and waned, I knew she felt safe and I know she knew she was loved.

I'm often surprised at how much gentleness and patience and compassion and soothing ability I apparently have as part of who I am that I'd just never seen or realized until I was caring for Mom full-time.

I never got excited about anything and always reassured Mom that everything was okay and she didn't need to apologize for or get upset about anything. I made sure Mom knew I wanted to do this and that I was happy to do it and that I loved her unconditionally. Because I was and I did. And I do.

There are moments of those last eight months that I won't forget. One was the morning Mom woke up around 9 am and sat up and I sat down on the bed beside her and held her hand and she asked me if I saw the two angels across the room.

Somehow I had the presence of mind to realize Mom was hallucinating, so I asked her to tell me about them and she gave me very detailed descriptions about where they were and what they looked like.

Another time we got up in the middle of the night so Mom could go to the bathroom and she demanded that I close the door so "that man can't see me." I did and when we got ready to go back to bed, Mom asked me where he was. I told her he'd gone upstairs.

Whatever it was that was on Mom's mind stayed a while, because when Mom woke up the next morning, she asked me where the man and the children were. I told her they were gone and it was just the two of us at the house. Mom accepted that and didn't ask about it again.

After a gallbladder infection in March and a hospitalization, Mom and I talked and she decided she didn't want to go back in the hospital again. I told Mom that was okay and that's what we'd do.

By this time, I realized Mom's congestive heart failure was worsening and I needed to make sure we had the medical help in place to deal with her end of life.

I don't know what happened with Mom's P.A., but he simply refused to accept that Mom was on her way to dying and I couldn't get him to do the things that needed to be done to ensure Mom's comfort and that it was as easy and painless for her as possible.

At that point I switched to another doctor in the group and he and I agreed to manage Mom's congestive heart failure (parameters that he gave me about weight gain and temporary increases in her diuretics to pull the excess fluid off) at home.

He told Mom and me both that she was in the dying process and the body was beginning its shutdown process. I think Mom and I both - or at least I - already knew that, but I was thankful that he recognized it and talked with both of us about it.

By the end of May, Mom had lost the concentration to work on puzzles anymore, so I began coloring activities that we did together and I started reading a lot aloud to her from books and from the Bible.

By July, Mom had slowed down and weakened considerably. Except for a surprise burst of energy one day in the middle of the month, Mom spent a lot of time sleeping. I'd try to get Mom out and keep her moving as much as she felt like it, but everything tired her out very easily, and she just didn't have a whole lot of energy.

We'd talk a lot and Mom worried near the end about me and being a burden on me. I told Mom she wasn't a burden on me and I was with her all the way through this process and I'd be waiting to see her in the resurrection. I told her I wasn't going anywhere and it was going to be all right.

Mom had been complaining of continuous shoulder and neck pains since getting a cold in early May. Those worsened over the next two and a half months, but I didn't see any heart distress. I knew Mom's heart and the aortic valve were wearing out, but she didn't specifically identify her heart as being the source of pain until one day in early August.

I called home health and they told me to take Mom to the hospital if she was having chest pains. I told them Mom didn't want to go to the hospital and we'd agreed on that. They sent hospice out that day and Mom was admitted to hospice for heart disease.

I received the hospice kit the next morning and Mom had a major heart attack that night. I recognized that Mom was having a heart attack because I'd been with my dad when he'd had one of his heart attacks. After some morphine, the pain subsided. The hospice nurse came out and said Mom's vital signs looked okay, but to keep a close eye on her through the night.

After the nurse left, Mom and I sat hugging each other on the couch for a while until she told me she was tired and wanted to go to the recliner to sleep.

Mom slept for the majority of the next two days, although she woke up intermittently to eat, drink, and go to the bathroom. Mom had lost a lot of mobility with the heart attack and the hospice nurse that came Friday suggested a different walker and a hospital bed, which I ordered and were delivered on Monday.

By the middle of the next week, Mom had regained a little strength and she was able to walk with my help to the bathroom and back for baths and when she needed to use the bathroom. I stayed close by Mom all week and I read and we talked non-stop when she was awake. Although Mom didn't know who I was, she trusted me and I knew she was glad I was there.

My sister came to town Friday afternoon and Mom recognized her as soon as she walked in the door and was glad to see her. Even though I was sitting right there, Mom talked to my sister about me in the third person and wanted to know where I was and if I was coming to visit too.

The next morning when Mom woke up, my sister and I both walked in, and Mom knew us both.

Mom was happy to see us, alert, and had a decent amount of energy.

We were able to spend a lot of the day outside talking and laughing about a lot of good times in our lives. My one concern that day was Mom's lack of urine output, even though she was eating and drinking normally.

By the time Mom went to the memory-care community, she had some urinary incontinence – she'd feel the urge to go, but couldn't get to the bathroom in time – and had been wearing "adult panties," as I called them since then.

After she came to live with me, Mom was even more incontinent – especially when the diuretics were increased to deal with her congestive heart failure – and we often had multiple clothing and underwear changes a day and always in the morning when she first got up.

So for Mom to stay bone-dry all day was alarming to me. After we got Mom tucked in for the night, I told my sister I was concerned that Mom's kidneys were shutting down and we needed to keep an eye on that.

When Mom woke up bone-dry the next morning – although still happy, still alert, and still knowing who we were and glad that we were there – I decided to call the hospice nurse.

When the nurse got there, I told her what was going on and what my concerns were. She checked Mom out and said everything looked good and looked healthy and happy, so it didn't seem like a problem yet. The nurse said that she'd stop back by that night and if Mom was still not outputting a lot of urine, she'd put a catheter in to stimulate the bladder into normal functioning.

Mom and we ate breakfast and enjoyed a nice round of conversation. After Mom ate and we talked a little while longer, Mom said she was tired and thought she'd take a little nap.

That was Mom's normal pattern, so I covered her up and Deb and I told Mom we loved her and Mom told us she loved us and we kissed her and let her get some sleep.

When Mom awoke a few hours later, we were in the room and we could immediately see that her whole disposition had changed.

Mom looked at us, we thought angrily, but in hindsight, I think she was having another heart attack and was scared.

We gave Mom a little yogurt to eat because she said she was hungry and tried to get her to drink some water, but she pushed the cup away.

Mom then said to us "I guess they're going to throw me out now." This seemed like a random statement, but we both sat with Mom and held her hands and told her she was home and we were with her and nobody was going to throw her out. I got a photo album with family pictures out and turned the pages for Mom. The only one of us Mom recognized was Daddy.

Mom then told me she was in a lot of pain - she didn't have the cold, clammy sweating nor was the color drained out of her face like the first heart attack she'd had - and I asked where the pain was.

Mom pointed across her back and chest and I decided to give her a dose of morphine, since that was what hospice told me to give her for chest pains (it relaxes the heart) and respiratory distress (it slows the breathing down to normal).

I could give Mom up to two doses at a time, but I started with one. Mom looked at Daddy's picture again, closed her eyes, and continued turning the blank pages of the photo album.

Mom never woke up again from that sleep, but we were by her side all the way, talking to her, making sure she knew we all loved her, reading to her, singing to her, holding her hands and rubbing her head and her arms, to the last breath.

Mom died comfortably and peacefully on August 14, 2012 and she now rests awaiting a resurrection to complete healing inside and out.

Chapter 4: Lessons to Pass On

There are a lot of books out there on caregiving for loved ones with dementias and Alzheimer's. What I found from the few I tried to read was a lot of convoluted repetitive theory, but no practical application. I waded through the torrent of words with no more knowledge of how Mom and I were going to do this in practical terms than I started with.

And that is why I wrote this book. To give you the practical application of the lessons I learned in a hands-on and accessible way, so you have the big-picture guide that I basically had to figure out by myself to make sure your loved ones get the best care possible.

- Proactively and thoroughly educate yourself, your loved one(s), and your doctor(s)

  I spent a lot of time each time Mom had a diagnosis getting a complete confirmation and picture of what she and I were dealing with and what outcomes were expected.

For example, as Mom's Lewy Body dementia symptoms got more pronounced, I researched the symptoms and realized that she had Lewy Body dementia in addition to vascular dementia and Alzheimer's Disease. (Lewy Body dementia can't be confirmed definitively except by a post-mortem examination of the brain, but the symptoms are so unique, it's easy to diagnose it in life.)

This is important, especially from a medication standpoint, since many of the drugs used to manage the symptoms of dementias and Alzheimer's Disease are prescribed "off-label" (meaning the drug is intended to treat a different disease) and I found that a lot of the drugs that were suggested for Mom had specific warnings that they were not to be given to elderly dementia patients.

Here are a couple of practical examples:

- Abilify, which is now being advertised, in an "off-label" use for the general public, as an anti-depressant, is manufactured to treat schizophrenia. It has the "no elderly dementia" warning on the drug's fact sheet. Yet, Mom's P.A. wanted me to fill a prescription for it.

- SeroquelXR, which is an anti-psychotic medication, should be carefully monitored when used with people suffering from Lewy Body dementia, since about half of the people with Lewy Body dementia who are given anti-psychotic medications to control the hallucinations are highly sensitive to them and other problems and issues can arise from that.

There several websites that you
may want to bookmark and use
as day-to-day guides for
questions and answers:

- Lewy Body Dementia
  Association -
  http://www.lbda.org/
- Vascular (Multi-Infarct)
  Dementia:
  http://www.nlm.nih.gov/med
  lineplus/ency/article/000746.
  htm
- Alzheimer's Disease:
  http://www.nia.nih.gov/alzh
  eimers/publication/alzheimer
  s-disease-fact-sheet
- Congestive Heart Failure:
  http://www.nanocorthx.com/
  Articles/WhatisHeartFailure.p
  df
- The Dying Process:
  http://bentonhospice.org/ind
  ex.php?action=patients.stage
  s

There are many other resources out there. Use them.

- This is a full-time job and the quality of your job performance will affect the quality of your loved one(s) life/lives

  It took a while for me to be consciously aware that taking care of Mom was my full-time job and how well and how much I applied myself to do the job right for her had a direct correlation to what the quality of the rest of her life was going to be.

  While love and obligation are part of the reasons we choose to care for our loved ones through the last years of our lives, we also need to approach this stage of our lives with the same commitment to excellence, to doing what it takes to get the job done, to succeeding that we do to paid employment.

Whether you are being compensated – I was not (and didn't want to be – Mama and Daddy had done this with no pay for my sisters and me when we were babies and completely helpless and dependent on them for everything, so, for me, this was just doing the same for both of them when they needed it) and most of us are not – or not for the care you're providing to your loved ones, you are performing the same job and have the same responsibilities as a chief executive officer (CEO) of a corporation.

You are solely responsible for the big picture of finances, health, and legal issues for your loved one(s). How well you fulfill those responsibilities will determine the "success" of your tenure.

- Be an advocate for your loved one(s)

As our loved one(s) get older, weaker, and the dementias

progress, they will be less able to communicate well with us and others. It's important that you stand in the gap for them by listening to them, knowing them well enough to know what they are trying to communicate, and making sure that you communicate their wishes clearly to financial, health, and legal professionals.

That means you have to be actively engaged and involved all the time. Remember that these professionals see your loved one(s) sporadically and for short periods of time, but you're with them all the time and are aware of subtle or slow changes or issues that emerge that these professionals may not see.

It's up to you, then, to make sure those changes and issues are addressed. And don't stop until it is clear that you've been heard and understood. It doesn't mean being rude or abrasive, but it means standing your ground and being persistent.

- Be willing to fire your loved one(s) doctor(s)

No matter how good the relationship has been between a doctor and a patient, doctors are still human and occasionally that humanness gets in the way of their ability to provide the right treatment.

For example, Mom's P.A. is a wonderful man and was excellent in treating her until it was clear that she was reaching the terminal stage of congestive heart failure and the dementias and Alzheimer's Disease. Then he shut down and would not listen to me nor would he do the things we needed, healthcare-wise (palliative care and hospice), to make sure Mom was comfortable and the dying process was as easy and painless for her as possible.

I don't think he could accept the fact that Mom was dying and that he couldn't do anything else to stop that, so he refused to accept it. It was that simple. And while I understood that, it wasn't helping Mom, so I had to fire him as Mom's doctor and hire a doctor who could deal with it and help Mom out.

If you have to fire a doctor, try to have the conversation with him or her about why and make sure it's an objective conversation instead of an emotional one. I was not able to have that conversation with Mom's P.A. because he'd already shut me out, but I made sure that the doctor I hired next got the message and passed it on to him.

- Be sure to include your loved one(s) in all discussions about them

One of the things that would drive me crazy while taking care of Mom was when she was sitting in the room and whoever we were seeing would talk to me and pretend like Mom wasn't even there. That was a respect and a dignity issue for me and I would not allow it.

Even if Mom didn't completely understand or hear all of the conversations, I always would make a point of turning to her and talking to her and including her in every single conversation. And the other person or people involved would follow my lead.

This is a walking-in-someone-else's-shoes point. These diseases are isolating enough. Throw a profound hearing loss on top of that and the isolation factor increases exponentially. Invisibility is even further isolation. Think about how that would affect you. That's how it affects your loved one(s).

- Give yourself and your time to your loved one(s) to show you love them and you care about them

There's a lot of "stuff" that has to be done for our loved one(s) suffering from dementias and health issues. It's the same kind of stuff that parents have to do for babies.

Bathing, feeding, dressing, changing, and handling crises, along with laundry, food preparation, doing the dishes, cleaning up messes, and cleaning the house is part of what we do day in and day out.

But all of that, in the end, is just busy work that has to be done, but it doesn't require love or affection.

I hope each of you reading this were fortunate enough to have, as children, snuggle time each day with your loved one(s).

I hope all of you reading this were fortunate enough to have,

as children, play time each day
with your loved one(s)s.

I hope each one of you reading
this were fortunate enough to
have, as children, reading time
with your loved one(s).

I hope each one of you reading
this was fortunate enough to
have, as children, a lot of hugs,
a lot of "I love you's," and the
gift of being tucked into bed by
your loved one(s) each night.

This is what I'm talking about
when I say that you need to
make sure you take the time to
give and show your love to your
loved one(s) every day.

Remember what that meant to
you as a child and how, no
matter how good or bad the day
had gone, you knew you were
loved and you knew you were
cared about and you knew you

mattered and you knew you were safe.

These diseases turn the tables faster than usual in the aging process on the parent-child relationship. You become the parent and your loved one(s) become the child.

Treat your loved one(s) the way, if you had a great childhood, you were treated, or, if you didn't have a great childhood, the way you would have wanted to have been treated.

I always told Mom that I was going to do my best to make sure her second childhood was better than her first one. And it was through this time of connecting, holding, talking, reading, and tucking in that I did my best during each day to keep that promise to Mom.

- Stay with your loved one(s) when they are hospitalized

  Hospitalizations are difficult on elderly people. When they suffer from dementias and Alzheimer's Disease, hospitalizations are traumatic for them because of the constant activity and the influx of strangers day and night.

  Having you there, both during the day and night, gives them a familiar face and security. It also enables you to advocate and be involved with what's going on.

  One of the biggest problems that can arise from hospitalizations is medication changes.

  The doctors seeing your loved one(s) are not their regular doctors (most hospitals use hospitalists - who are doctors on staff exclusively at the hospital - now for patient care).

Additionally, if there is a systemic problem (cardiac, endocrine, gastrointestinal, etc.), a doctor who specializes in that system will be involved in treatment.

And they will discharge your loved one(s) with the medication changes they made in the hospital and your loved one(s) regular doctor(s) will not be aware of that.

It's important for you to schedule a follow-up appointment with your loved one(s) regular doctor(s) as soon as possible after your loved one(s) are discharged from the hospital to review the medications and ensure that is the regimen that he or she wants to continue.

Often patients are released with medications they were taking for an acute problem, but do not need to take any longer or take in that dosage long-term.

If the hospital room has an empty bed in the room, the staff will let you sleep there. If not, there is usually a chair that will enable you to sleep right beside the bed of your loved one(s) at night.

This will be one of the greatest gifts of love you can provide.

Be aware that hospital stays always mean setbacks for your loved one(s). When you bring them home, try to get back into the quiet, normal routine you've established there as quickly as possible. This will help your loved one(s) settle down and feel safe and secure again.

• Make sure hospital discharges include home health agency follow-up at home

Usually what causes hospitalizations is not a direct symptom of the dementias and Alzheimer's disease. A health crisis

- pneumonia, heart issues, kidney issues, etc. - are usually the reason patients are hospitalized, so it's important to have home health nursing care after your loved one(s) gets home to ensure that the issues are stabilized.

In addition, home health agencies have physical therapists, speech therapists, and occupational therapists who can help you and your loved one(s) have as much quality of life and support as is possible.

• Do the research on home health agencies and remember that you get to decide who you want to use

Most hospitals partner with a home health agency and will try to get you to use their partner for your loved one(s) care.

You do not have to use their partner.

Go ahead and do your research early and know which health care agency you want to use when the time comes.

Also, be aware that most health care agencies offer at a minimum, home health and hospice services. If you can find a home health agency that offers palliative care – this is the stage between home health and hospice – that is your best option to ensure continuous medical support for your loved one(s).

You should also be aware that you don't have to use the same health care agency for all three of these types of care. Again, it's important that you do the research and know who you want to provide these three levels of care for your loved one(s).

I learned that in the health care agency setting, each level of care is a separate group under separate management and the quality of care among groups can be like night and day.

For example, the home health care Mom had was awesome. She had great nurses (and continuity) and a great physical therapist. The palliative care continued with this staff and was superb.

My initial contact with this health agency's hospice (as well as another health agency's hospice) was awful. However, when it came time to switch Mom from palliative care to hospice, the hospice nurse showed up with the home health nurse and said it was time to switch and I didn't have the time to advocate for still other health agency whose hospice care had been highly recommended to me.

However, the majority of the first week of hospice care Mom was under was so bad - and the complete opposite of what the same health agency's home health's care had been - that I put a call into Mom's doctor to have him write the order for the new hospice group when he got back in town that following Monday.

That Friday, a hospice nurse came and talked with Mom, me and my sister for quite a while after he'd checked Mom out.

I asked him if he was normally a home health nurse and he looked surprised and answered "yes." It was that different.

The hospice change never took place because Mom started the dying process on Sunday afternoon, but the Friday nurse said he'd take care of Mom for the rest of the time she was in hospice when I asked if he would, and he did and that was the only saving grace for that group.

But I would never recommend that hospice group to anyone else.

- Respite care is a bad idea

  All the traditional books on the market about caregiving urge the caregivers to take time for themselves and take advantage of respite care. This is a bad idea from a practical standpoint.

  One of the most important things you can provide for your loved one(s) who are suffering from dementias and Alzheimer's Disease is routine, security, and safety. The littlest changes can rock their worlds.

  Imagine yourself being confused, having hallucinations, and not being able to hear suddenly being put into a group environment (the other option is hospitalization and we already know what that does) with all new and strange people, routines, and things going on. How would you react?

As a caregiver, you committed to this and when it's over, you'll have time to recover and take care of yourself.

But while you're on the job, this is tantamount to abandoning your responsibility.

And I know how much respite care is debated in the community, but ask yourself this question in terms of fulfilling the circle of life: did your parents get respite care when you and your siblings were babies? Would they have ever thought about it, no matter how tired, how exhausted, and, yes, how exasperated at times they were?

The other issue with respite care is whether you would really be able to relax and enjoy yourself while you're away from your loved one(s).

I knew that I knew Mom and I knew how to take care of her and make sure everything was okay, and I frankly didn't believe nor trust that anyone else could or would do that for her. I was the one mostly-familiar and safe person in Mom's life and I refused to take that small sliver of comfort and trust away from her.

I have heard this is radical thinking. I have had people strongly disagree with it. But I stand by it. I made plenty of mistakes while taking care of Mom, but this is one of the things I know I got right.

You have to remember in this scenario that it's not really about you. It's about your loved one(s) and what they need and what's best for them is the only option. You'll be okay. They won't. It's that simple.

- Be patient with everybody, including yourself

I've never been one of the world's most patient people. The person I've always been the most impatient with is myself. That changed, for the better, while I took care of Mom. Did I screw up? Absolutely! Are there things that I wish I had known or had done differently? You bet!

But I learned that my reactions to things affected Mom for better or for worse, so I learned to be patient with myself and with her.

I'm a big-picture person, so I don't tend to sweat the details so much, but there's a lot of detail to pay attention to as a caregiver.

But my focus was always on Mom and making sure she didn't feel bad about the things out of her control, that she didn't feel like a burden, and that she knew I loved her and whatever happened, it was okay and we'd see it through together.

Ironically, it was very different from a lot of Mom's parenting of me, but I realize that she parented us kids the way she was parented and because of her lifelong issues with anxiety, she was on the edge most of the time, not because she wanted to be, but because she didn't know any differently. But regardless of Mom's parenting style, we kids knew that she loved us, if not all the time, most of the time.

- Help is not always help – even though that's the intent behind it

There's help and there's *help*. A lot of people, even family, want to help, but they actually end up making more work for you, so you realize that going it alone is better for you and for your loved one(s).

That's okay. There are nice ways to handle this without cutting yourself off at the knees in case the first kind of help is all you have available when you absolutely need extra hands.

But don't feel bad about admitting it and doing something about.

In the long run, it's going to make things easier for you and your loved one(s).

- Start a personal blog and write things down

  This is a way to capture memories, explain what you're seeing and experiencing and what your loved one(s) are going through. It's an excellent way to process things, to clarify things, and to settle things.

  And when your loved one(s) die, at some point, you will want to go back through the written record and you'll have it there when you're ready to do that.

- Prepare to miss your loved one(s) profoundly when they die and yet be thankful they are not suffering and that's a tough balancing act

The day Mom started her death sleep I had prayed that morning and cried as I asked God to have mercy on Mom and give her rest because she didn't have any quality of life left.

God answered that prayer, just as He had when I finally was able to pray that my dad not have to suffer anymore.

But even though I knew Mom's pain and suffering were over and I was thankful for that, I missed her more than I ever imagined I would. I grieved...I'm still grieving, which is one of the reasons I'm writing this book.

I did realize later that I was missing the person that Mom was before all the illnesses, before all the dementias, and the Alzheimer's Disease, and that was the person I was grieving the loss of.

It's better today than it was a month ago and the month before that and the month before that, but there's always a void that can never be filled up again in this life. And it takes time to process and accept it internally no matter how much you've done it intellectually.

- Make the experience count

  I'll tell you so far how I'm making the experience count. You will certainly think of more. Whatever, they are, make them happen.

  The first thing I did was include this experience on my resume. As I said earlier, this is a CEO position, so it made sense to include it as part of what I bring to the table with a potential employer.

  The second thing I did was write a memoir about our family, starting with my parents' childhoods and continuing through to Mom's death.

I wanted to capture all of that while it was at the forefront of my mind. The book is titled "Fields of Gold: A Love Story of Two Orphans, Their Union, and the Children They Adopted" and can be purchased from Amazon.

I have plans, if there's enough profit from the book, to start a foundation in my parents' names to provide help to seniors with medical equipment, prescription payment help, food and utilities if they need it, and medical advocacy.

I've heard about and seen too many elderly people either without family or family who was far away or didn't care all alone and also those without enough financial support to get what they need to be cared for. I won't solve all of the needs that are out there, but I will at least make an attempt to start.

I hope this has helped you.

The companion blog to this book is: http://goinggentleintothatgoodnight.com

You can subscribe to the blog to get updates as they are posted.

If you'd like to ask me any questions or more specific information I can help you with, please email me at goinggentleintothatgoodnight@gmail.com.

Best wishes to you and your loved one(s)!